7 secrets of abundant energy

 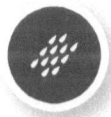     

Duane Alley

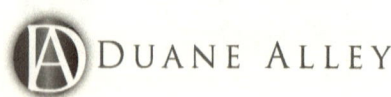
DUANE ALLEY

7 Secrets of Abundant Energy

Copyright © 2011 by Duane Alley – http://www.duanealley.com

All rights reserved. No part of this book may be produced or utilised in any form or by any means, electronic or mechanical, including photocopying, recording or by any information storage and retrieval system, without permission in writing from the Publisher.

Published 2011

Publisher: Performance Results Pty Ltd

Graphic Design & Layout: Mélissa Caron – Enki Communications – Go-Enki.com
Editor: Richard Burian – Enki Communications – Go-Enki.com

Health, Self Help

ISBN 978-0-9870571-2-9

For Sue Alley, my Mum.

An amazing example of all the energy

to keep going no matter what, always.

Thank you, love you. D

table of contents

About the author 9

1. Introduction 11

2. Abundance in Vibrant Breath 17

3. Abundance in Clean, Fresh Water 27

4. Abundance in Healthy, Vibrant Food 39

5. Abundance in Dynamic Exercise 51

6. Abundance in Restful Sleep 63

7. Abundance in Clear and Centred Mind 81

8. Abundance in Supportive Environment 91

9. Conclusion 103

about the author: Duane Alley

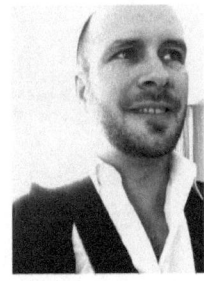

Trainer | Author | Speaker | Coach

Duane Alley spent the first 15 years of his professional life working with some of the biggest and fastest growing retail and franchise businesses in the country; he then spent 5 years as Head Trainer & Coach for one of the biggest Personal Development companies on the planet.

He has combined his extensive experience from the business world in delivering real world results with his success and study of personal development, rapid human change and shifting consciousness.

As a Master Trainer, Author, Speaker and Performance Coach he now works with businesses and entrepreneurs quickly and easily improve their businesses and make more money and with individuals, couples and families to make simple changes and take small steps to live better lives day by day.

Keep in touch:

- www.duanealley.com
- www.facebook.com/DuaneAlleyPage
- www.twitter.com/DuaneAlley
- www.youtube.com/DuaneAlley
- success@duanealley.com

1. introduction

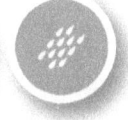

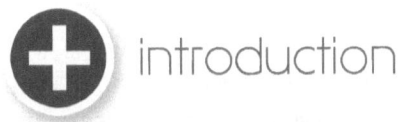

introduction

Over the last 5 years I have spent over 12,000 hours teaching, presenting and coaching people from different stages of life all over the world. I have delivered 12–14 hour days back to back for up to 7 days in 12 countries across 5 continents. One thing I do know is that the amount of ENERGY one has is crucial to success; and I'm not talking about pumped up caffeine pills or the "barely getting by, but I know I have to 'cause everyone's depending on me" martyr syndrome. I've seen enough of that to know it just doesn't work for the long term. And, let's face it, in this "life" thing – we want it to be long term.

The thing most people don't realise is they can have it LONG TERM, and it can be incredibly exciting and incredibly full. To pull it off though, you have to have real, honest to God energy; in abundance, my friends, with plenty left over. Because the truth is – you will always need more of it than you think.

I was a guest on a well known spiritual and personal development radio show – *The Aware Show* – from California a few years back and my great friend and host of the show, Lisa Garr, asked me something like, "so people are usually cup-half-empty or cup-half-full people, Duane. Which one are you?" Now, I know Lisa was expecting me to say "why, cup-half-full, of course". It's not what I said though. I was quiet for a moment and then responded, "Lisa, I never want half of anything. My cup is fully full – ALL the time." I truly believe that's what "full-*fill*-ment" means. Our lives were meant to be full, filled with passionate and purposeful experiences and relationships ALL The time. It is not just a good goal, but it is a divine birth right to be able to experience life at its fullest and enjoy the greatest levels of passion and abundance at every turn.

My mission is to help people live better lives every day. To help people create small shifts and learn simple lessons that will come together to create massive shifts in their results, their lives and the lives of those they love the most. This book and program then is about creating that level of energy in you, holding onto it and truly experiencing the abundance of it so you can live the passionate, powerful and purposeful life you were always meant to live.

It is absolutely true that the first secret to creating the greatest abundant resource of energy for life comes from living every day of your life with passion – passion for what you do, who you are and who you surround yourself with. Knowing the purpose of your existence and the difference you were meant to create for yourself and other people in the world. This book though is not about that. It's a whole separate topic. Because, truthfully – that's not the ONLY answer AND to get to the place of having the energy to find your passion and purpose, you still need to have the greatest amount of energy possible. Now THAT'S what *The 7 Secrets of Abundant Energy* is all about.

Too often, WAY too often I see people caught in what I call the "mindset trap", whereby something is not 100% in their life or it suddenly goes wrong and they immediately jump onto the next "mindset" or personal development training focussed on teaching them how to think or feel as if somehow that is the only thing that can be faulty in their lives. Please hear me out here – personal development is one of my greatest passions and joys – it helped lift me out of some very dark times and showed me the way to find my path and live the life I enjoy today. I have seen the incredible impact it can have on anyone's lives. I have also seen many students of it deluded into thinking that all they have to do is change their thinking and feeling and suddenly everything will be exactly as they want it. Unfortunately, there are a number of teachers in the field who promote just that. The reasons range from being that's what they learned and now they are just regurgitating and hoping that by teaching they will somehow be successful themselves. Bluntly and honestly – it's a good marketing ploy for many of these "teachers" (I use the word really loosely here). There was a recent spate of movies and programs that opened up the world of personal development to a whole new audience – I credit those movies for driving the learning out to a whole new group of people, BUT if I were to make my own follow-up movie to all of them I have often said in my own seminars, I would call it – *The Sequel: The Secret to Getting Off Your Arse and Doing Something About It*. Action is mandatory for success. Full stop. This book is about DOING things that will make a difference. When you want a result on a particular plane of existence you MUST operate in that plane. If you want emotional change – work emotionally. If you want a physical change of more energy – there has to be some work done in the physical plane. There'll be learning AND strategies to follow to ensure you get the result you are after.

There'll be a lot of moments that I refer to in my seminars as "Oh, Of Course!" moments. It's when you hear or see something and realise you know this somewhere in you already. I've heard many of my Personal Development friends call them "blinding flashes of the obvious". There'll also be some new information – take it in, sit with it for a while, try it on and see how it works for you. And of course inevitably there'll be those moments when you see something that's directly opposite to where you'd normally be thinking or acting. In those moments – please stay with me (and with the program) – again I ask you to try it on, see how the new thinking or behaving fits and sits with you. Most importantly, check out the results you get from it. Be open and you might very well be surprised by the result and it could lead to a paradigm shift you're going to be very happy with.

Okay – buckle up, strap in and let's roll...

Green Lights all the way!

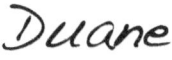

Duane Alley
Creator/Author, The 7 Secrets Series
DuaneAlley Training and DuaneAlley Coaching

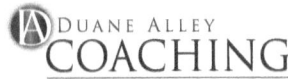 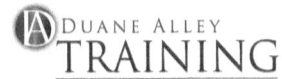

2. abundance in vibrant breath

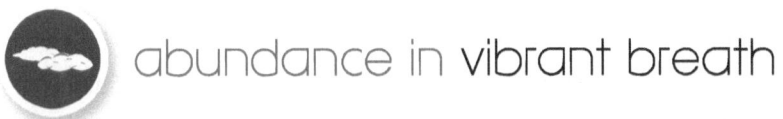 # abundance in vibrant breath

It is very well known that you can survive weeks without food. You can get by for days without water, but take away "breathing" and you won't even be around for minutes.

Breathing is a constant from birth to death, yet for the most part we pay little attention to it. Adults typically breathe between 12 and 20 times per minute when resting – children breathe faster. Breathing usually takes place one nostril at a time – this changes every 15 minutes to 3 hours depending on the person.

There are more metaphors that can be named here that link breath to life itself in many languages. The Hawai'ians thought breath was so important they named their home for it – "Ha" in Hawai'ian means "breath of life". In fact the only difference the ancient Hawai'ians saw between a living person and someone who just died is that the breath had left them. They reasoned then that our life-force must travel on the breath. Hawai'ian folk say that the "Wai" – from "Hawaii" means "life force".

Ancient knowledge and practices used conscious attention to breathing in many forms of meditation (e.g., yoga, Qi Gong, Tai Chi). In fact, learning one of these arts is a fundamental way to truly learn the art of "breathing for life". Every martial arts practitioner uses conscious breath control today. Breathing is one of the few bodily functions that can, within limits, be controlled both consciously and unconsciously. Every psychological, emotional, chemical and physiological state has a corresponding breathing pattern or quality. The way we breathe is so intrinsically linked to our nervous system that by bringing conscious attention to breathing you can access various energies and trigger different emotional states.

Breathing patterns are unique to individuals – changing not only with each person but also with each moment. The way you breathe when you are angry is different from when you are calm and peaceful; the way you breathe in the dentist's chair is different from the way you breathe when you are having an orgasm.

Let's talk pure physiology for a minute. Breathing is a complex mechanism and process that involves a number of levels and aspects. First, form structure and mechanics of breathing: the physical tension and muscular co-ordination involved. Posture is an important aspect of breathing. Good posture supports good breathing and good breathing supports good posture.

Imagine you have run a long race – you are exhausted and "gasping for air" in an attempt to recover. What do you do? You stand upright and stretch out your torso in order to support the most complete filling of your lungs – to get as much air into them as possible. The chemistry of breathing is also important; the exchange process of carbon dioxide (CO_2) and oxygen is the key chemical reaction that takes place from breathing. CO_2 controls the dilation and constriction of the smooth muscles that make up the walls of the arteries, intestines and bronchial vessels, it also sets the stage for oxygen delivery to the cells and among other things, it is critical in the control of the acid-alkaline balance in the body's blood chemistry. Breath control and awareness can adjust and regulate many bodily chemical reactions and have an impact on a host of biological factors vital to health and well-being.

On a subtler level and linked to all that you have read so far, breathing has a direct relationship with our energy level and also that quality of energy available to us. This is not some new age "guess" though; as mentioned, all martial arts teach methods of conscious breath control to bring on certain emotional states and access levels of energy and consciousness not normally activated in everyday life. This energy, in China is called CHI; Japan – KI; India –PRANA;

Latin – SPIRITUS (meaning the animating principal of life); In Hebrew – RUACH (meaning the breath within the breath). It is believed by many cultures that this is our vital life force energy.

So how do we use what we know?

The process is this:

Acceptance

Once you have new information, particularly if it is different to how you have thought or operated within the past, it is critical to "accept" that there is a different way of approaching things; a potentially new and different way to do things and therefore achieve different results that could be available to you. It is also equally important to accept that you might want to change your old habits for new ones in order to reach a better result.

Accept that you are intricately linked to the world around you by the breath you breathe in and the breath you breathe out. Accept that your breath is an ancient thing that gives you life and sustains your life force.

Awareness

Becoming "aware" is the first (and sometimes only) thing necessary for change. It is the crucial step to changing the results. You must become aware of where you are at and what you are doing. Aware of the new habits to be taken in and the new possibilities that will open up to you once you begin to act in new ways.

You can become aware of your surroundings by controlling and regulating your breathing. If you take any form of martial arts, yoga or tai chi, you will learn how to do this. For example, people who shoot know that they hit their target when their breathing is in complete harmony and they are at peace.

Activation

All the "thinking" done – it's time for "*real*-ising" – that is, making it happen in the real world – and putting into action what you know you need to do.

Once your breathing is in control, you are ready to act upon and realise your wishes.

Appreciate

Finally, as in all things, it is critical to "appreciate" what you have accomplished and be grateful for having achieved it. Even if it is one step forward on a long journey you are now one step further along the path and that is infinitely better than where you were before; even accepting that there could be change. Appreciation is the step we keep with us constantly; every change, improvement and moment of growth is a moment to appreciate what you have done and what you are "doing" even now. It is important to go as far as to reward yourself for the achievements. A great friend and teacher of mine, Clinton Swaine, used to teach his classes to "Celebrate All Achievements". This changed one day when he realised that it was not only the achievement of the goal that required reward but rather every step along the way was begging for recognition. He now teaches his students, "Celebrate Everything".

Be grateful and appreciate the fact that you can breathe air and that it sustains your life. Celebrate this fact and this connection that you have with everyone and everything living that is around you. You even have a connection with inanimate objects through your breath, as the oxygen you breathe in and the carbon dioxide you breathe out can turn iron to rust and copper green.

Where does this leave you right now? You have read and completed the "acceptance" bit; now it's time for awareness. Think where you are currently "at" with breathing consciously and how you use this fundamental mechanism for physical success to your own advantage.

Rate yourself below on a scale of 1-10.

1: I suck at this. Through to 10: I'm incredible at this.
If you scored yourself a "4" or below, then it's time to take some massive action in this area. You need a strategy to create change here.

❶ Where are you now?
○ 1 ○ 2 ○ 3 ○ 4 ○ 5 ○ 6 ○ 7 ○ 8 ○ 9 ○ 10

❷ Where do you want to be in 30 days?
○ 1 ○ 2 ○ 3 ○ 4 ○ 5 ○ 6 ○ 7 ○ 8 ○ 9 ○ 10

❸ Where do you want to be in 3 months?
○ 1 ○ 2 ○ 3 ○ 4 ○ 5 ○ 6 ○ 7 ○ 8 ○ 9 ○ 10

❹ Where do you want to be in 6 months?
○ 1 ○ 2 ○ 3 ○ 4 ○ 5 ○ 6 ○ 7 ○ 8 ○ 9 ○ 10

❺ Where do you want to be in 12 months?
○ 1 ○ 2 ○ 3 ○ 4 ○ 5 ○ 6 ○ 7 ○ 8 ○ 9 ○ 10

❻ What aspects do you want to learn, change, grow, develop?

_____
_____

❼ How do you want to do that?

_____
_____

❽ What impact will that have on your life and/or the lives of those you love most?

_____
_____

❾ What is your plan? (Include names, dates, actions.)

_____
_____

❿ The first thing I need to do to make this happen is...

_____
_____

⓫ I'm going to do this when?

_____
_____

⓬ To whom or how am I going to be held accountable...

_____
_____

13 Today I will...

_____

_____

14 This week I will...

_____

_____

15 I'm ready to do this because...

_____

_____

That's it: plan set. Now it's time for you to put it in motion. If you have any work to do there, then it needs to be done and the momentum built. Do not move on to the next part until you have done something actively and positively towards shifting your personal outcome in this area. You don't have to have achieved your ultimate goal – just make sure you have a plan and that plan is already in play through your own actions.

When you are ready, let's get to the next secret. The secrets of...

3. abundance in clean, fresh water

abundance in clean, fresh water

Water makes up more than two thirds of the weight of a human body – without it humans would die in a few days. The human brain is made up of 75% water. Blood is 83%, the lungs 90%. A mere 2% drop in our body's water supply can trigger signs of dehydration: fuzzy short-term memory, trouble with basic math, difficulty focussing on small print (e.g. computer screen). Mild dehydration is one of the most common causes of daytime fatigue. Studies have estimated that a minimum of 75% of people in the UK, USA or Australia have mild, chronic dehydration.

Dehydration is when the body is not getting as much water and fluids as it should. Not drinking enough water or losing too much fluid can cause it. Infants and children are at higher risk of dehydration than adults as they have a smaller body weight and higher use of water and electrolytes. Those who are suffering from illnesses and the elderly are also at higher risk.

You can be mildly, moderately or severely dehydrated; when severe, dehydration is a life-threatening emergency.

Water is the most essential element, next to air, to our survival. Water is truly everywhere yet it is still taken for granted. Water is also one of the four ancient elements from ancient Greek philosophy, the Indian Panchamahabhuta and the Chinese system of cosmology known as Wu Xing. Water is associated with both emotion and intuition. Water is also associated with the ancient belief in the four humours, of which water was the phlegmatic one. Water was stoic, patient and apathetic. "As impassive as the ocean," goes the old saying. It is also associated in this lore with the brain, the feminine and the western point of the compass. In the Indian tradition water is thought to be feelings, intuition and imagination.

In the Zodiac, those who are born under the signs of Cancer, Scorpio and Pisces have dominant water personalities. They can be emotional, deep, nurturing, empathetic, sympathetic, imaginative and intuitive; as well as sentimental, sensitive and irrational.

Water makes its manifestation in rivers, oceans, lakes, wells, rain, fog, ice and snow. The dolphin, turtle, frog and all types of fish personify the element of water and in mythology there are creatures such as the mermaid, Naiad and sea serpent which are of the water as well.

The body CANNOT work without water – all cell and organ functions that make up our entire anatomy and physiology depend on water for their functioning. Water:

- serves as a lubricant

- is the basis of saliva

- forms fluids that surround joints

- regulates body temperature and perspiration

- is the best detox agent; moves waste through the intestinal tract; alleviates constipation

- regulates the metabolism

We most often notice the effects of dehydration (hypo-hydration) rather than the fact that we are correctly hydrated (have enough water). This is when the body doesn't have enough water to carry out its normal functions. The effects of dehydration are often insidious – you do not know they are happening or even that you have become dehydrated. This is how so many people live their lives constantly in a state of mild dehydration. Some symptoms include: a dry or sticky mouth, low or no urine output or concentrated urine that is dark yellow, not producing tears, sunken eyes, markedly sunken fontanels in an infant, lethargy or even coma (in severe dehydration). Millions of ordinary people die of dehydration each year. Even a small reduction in body fluids and electrolytes (lost along with the water when you dehydrate) leads to lower circulating blood-volume. As a result, your heart has to pump harder to maintain adequate blood-flow to your vital organs and you are less able to control your blood pressure, distribute nutrients and eliminate waste. Because you have less blood-volume you are also less able to dissipate heat through perspiration, therefore increasing your core body temperature and therefore leading to potential heat exhaustion and heat stroke.

Major causes of dehydration: diarrhoea, exercise, fever, increased urination, long airplane flights (the air on planes can be drier than the Sahara Desert), hot sunny climates and burns. You need to replace this water that you are losing otherwise you create a water deficit or dehydration, which is the elimination of more water and body salts that you are replenishing. Some water will come from the food you eat – the rest has to be consumed as liquid.

The amount of water that you should drink on a daily basis is a widely debated issue. The Mayo Clinic says that it is more about "replacement" than any form of prescription of quantity. Often it is said to drink 8x8 ounce glasses a day. It's a good model, but not really applicable to everyone and not backed up by much scientific research. An average person loses around 2.5L of water through just regular breathing, perspiration and elimination (roughly 10 cups) – this is before you even think about mowing the lawn, working out at the gym or doing the housework. The Mayo Clinic recommends at least 2L per day in addition to your regular diet, whereas the Institute of Medicine says that men should look to around 13 cups while women to 9 cups. The recommendations don't take into account individuals or individual circumstances – in certain cases; you may need to drink much more.

Perhaps the best recommendation is to continuously make a conscious effort to keep yourself hydrated and to make water your beverage of choice. Drink twice as much as it takes to quench your thirst.

When working with Private Clients on weight issues I always start with water intake. We start by eliminating other liquids and replacing with clean, fresh water only and radically increasing the amount. This is always because they are not consuming anywhere near an adequate amount. It's not just Clients working on controlling weight who I get to increase water – generally at some stage during any Coaching work I will suggest or impose this change. Water is essential for correct physical and mental functioning. You are not going to get the best results unless you are properly hydrated. I usually suggest 1L of fresh clean water for every 20KG of body weight and in most adults this comes with a minimum of 4L unless they are a very small person. Excess water just flows out without any problems. What I always tell them and they always find is that the more you start to drink, the thirstier you will find yourself being and the more you will enjoy water. This is because the body has been in a state of constant hypo-hydration (think of it like a water famine). Once your body realises you are giving it water in abundance, it can finally move from freaking out and keeping everything running on minimum to asking for what it really needs and wants.

Something more people are recognising is that hunger signals are often misinterpreted thirst signals – another cause of people becoming overweight. They are eating when they don't need to because they are actually thirsty. Double wammy. They end up storing excess fat and don't get the water they need to eliminate the fat.

The strategy I start my Coaching Clients on is simple:

a) **drink water** – only water – water with anything else in it is not water (with the exception of real lime, lemon or chlorophyll)

b) **do not count litres** – instead use the same size bottle and count bottles – once you get used to consuming x number of bottles a day just increase the size of the bottle – psychological trick but it works

c) **drink first thing after waking** – this is from the *7 Minute Secrets* also and one of my inspirations for putting it in that program

d) **drink between breakfast and lunch**

e) **drink between lunch and dinner**

f) **drink after dinner but not too late** or you'll be waking up to go to the toilet all night

You are automatically having 4 bottles of water without much effort – now just make any incidental drink water too and you are on your way to repaying your water debt and posting a credit balance on the ledger too.

So how do we use what we know?

The process is this:

Acceptance

Once you have new information, particularly if it is different to how you have thought or operated within the past, it is critical to "accept" that there is a different way of approaching things; a potentially new and different way to do things and therefore achieve different results that could be available to you. It is also equally important to accept that you might want to change your old habits for new ones in order to reach a better result.

Once you have understood that water is necessary for the proper functioning of your body, it's time to accept a new way of approaching it. Many people don't drink water because they simply haven't gotten used to it yet. You may hear the argument a lot that you don't "like" water. But once you accept that this is necessary and start drinking it, after a while there will be no turning back.

Awareness

Becoming "aware" is the first (and sometimes only) thing necessary for change. It is the crucial step to changing the results. You must become aware of where you are at and what you are doing. Aware of the new habits to be taken in and the new possibilities that will open up to you once you begin to act in new ways.

Be aware of how the water you drink changes you. Feel it cleansing any impurities in your body. Especially if you live in a city and walk around all day in the pollution, when you get a drink of water imagine it flushing the toxins from your body. When you get home, make yourself a tall glass of water with ice and drink it while relaxing on a hot summer day. Add a slice of lemon if you want. Be aware of the bubbles floating to the top of the glass, providing you with air as well as water. When you go out hiking, ask a ranger where you can get a drink of fresh, mountain spring water and become aware of the land, the earth, the sky and the entire cosmos when you drink it.

Activation

All the "thinking" done – it's time for "*real*-ising" – that is, making it happen in the real world – and putting into action what you know you need to do.

When you've come to terms with the necessity of abundant water in your life, then you can realise it. But water wherever you go. Try every different type you can find. Become a connoisseur of water like some people do with wine. Drink carbonated, plain and tap water. Try and compare all the water you find on your travels. Learn about the properties of minerals in natural water like iron, phosphorous and sulphites and how they can help you improve your mind and body.

Appreciate

Finally, as in all things, it is critical to "appreciate" what you have accomplished and be grateful for having achieved it. Even if it is one step forward on a long journey you are now one step further along the path and that is infinitely better than where you were before; even accepting that there could be change. Appreciation is the step we keep with us constantly; every change, improvement and moment of growth is a moment to appreciate what you have done and what you are "doing" even now. It is important to go as far as to reward yourself for the achievements. A great friend and teacher of mine, used to teach his classes to "Celebrate All Achievements". This changed one day when he realised that it was not only the achievement of the goal that required reward but rather every step along the way was begging for recognition. He now teaches his students, "Celebrate Everything".

Appreciate all the gifts that come in the form of water all over the planet. Appreciate that you are now healing your body through the power of water; one of the four ancient elements.

Where does this leave you right now? You have read and completed the "acceptance" bit; now it's time for awareness. Think where you are currently "at" with breathing consciously and how you use this fundamental mechanism for physical success to your own advantage.

Rate yourself below on a scale of 1-10.

1: I suck at this. Through to 10: I'm incredible at this.
If you scored yourself a "4" or below, then it's time to take some massive action in this area. You need a strategy to create change here.

❶ Where are you now?
○ ○ ○ ○ ○ ○ ○ ○ ○ ○
1   2   3   4   5   6   7   8   9   10

❷ Where do you want to be in 30 days?
○ ○ ○ ○ ○ ○ ○ ○ ○ ○
1   2   3   4   5   6   7   8   9   10

❸ Where do you want to be in 3 months?
○ ○ ○ ○ ○ ○ ○ ○ ○ ○
1   2   3   4   5   6   7   8   9   10

❹ Where do you want to be in 6 months?
○ ○ ○ ○ ○ ○ ○ ○ ○ ○
1   2   3   4   5   6   7   8   9   10

❺ Where do you want to be in 12 months?
○ ○ ○ ○ ○ ○ ○ ○ ○ ○
1   2   3   4   5   6   7   8   9   10

❻ What aspects do you want to learn, change, grow, develop?

_____

_____

7 How do you want to do that?

_____
_____

8 What impact will that have on your life and/or the lives of those you love most?

_____
_____

9 What is your plan? (Include names, dates, actions.)

_____
_____

10 The first thing I need to do to make this happen is...

_____
_____

11 I'm going to do this when?

_____
_____

12 To whom or how am I going to be held accountable...

_____
_____

13 Today I will...

_____
_____

14 This week I will...

_____

_____

15 I'm ready to do this because...

_____

_____

That's it: plan set. Now it's time for you to put it in motion. If you have any work to do there, then it needs to be done and the momentum built. Do not move on to the next part until you have done something actively and positively towards shifting your personal outcome in this area. You don't have to have achieved your ultimate goal – just make sure you have a plan and that plan is already in play through your own actions.

When you are ready, let's get to the next secret. The secrets of...

4. abundance in healthy, vibrant food

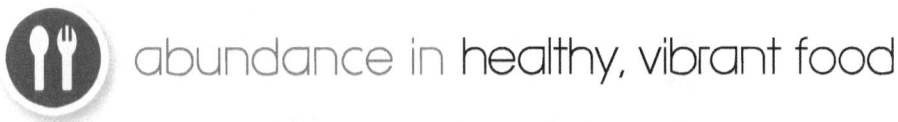# abundance in healthy, vibrant food

There are thousands of diets registered with the national diet association in the USA – this only goes to prove the inefficacy (and inadequacy) of most diets. Actually, there are more eating plans today than ever before – so much information – what do you do?

Before we talk about it, here's some history of the discoveries of the importance of food:

c. 475BC The Greek philosopher Anaxagoras deduces the existence of nutrients when he states that food is absorbed by the human body and therefore contains (what he called) *homeomerics* (generative components).

c. 400BC Hippocrates says, "Let food be your medicine and medicine be your food."

1500s Scientist and artist Leonardo da Vinci compared metabolism to a burning candle.

1747 Dr. James Lind, a physician in the British navy, performed the first scientific nutrition experiment, discovering that lime juice saved sailors who had been at sea for years from scurvy, a deadly and painful bleeding disorder. The discovery was ignored for years, after which British sailors became known as "limeys". The essential vitamin C within limes would not be recognised by scientists until the 1930s.

1770   Antoine Lavoisier, the "Father of Nutrition and Chemistry" discovered the details of metabolism, demonstrating that the oxidation of food is the source of body heat.

Early 1900s   Carl Von Voit and Max Rubner independently measure caloric energy expenditure in different species of animals, applying principles of physics to nutrition.

1912   Casmir Funk coined the term vitamin, a vital factor in the diet, from the words "vital" and "amine", because these unknown substances preventing scurvy, beriberi, and pellagra, were thought then to be derived from ammonia.

1913   Elmer V. McCollum discovered the first vitamins, fat-soluble vitamin A, and water-soluble vitamin B (in 1915; now known to be a complex of several water-soluble vitamins) and names vitamin C as the then-unknown substance preventing scurvy.

1936   Eugene Floyd Dubois shows that work and school performance are both related to caloric intake.

2002   Study shows the relationship between nutrition and violent behaviour.

So, back to the diets and eating plans... What do we do?

Of all the studies and new books that have been and are being released there is a common theme: the more natural and less processed a food is – the better off we are and the healthier the food is for us. Less processed food is food that is either eaten raw or cooked. Much of the food that you can find in grocery stores and supermarkets is far from natural. Many of them are made with a variety of synthetically created chemicals in laboratories, which are often not able to be assimilated properly by the body. Food is best eaten raw or cooked. Additionally, many of the books and plans out there are entirely prescriptive, meaning they tend to dictate a particular plan or style of food that is right for everyone. As humans though, we are not "one size fits all".

Here's another idea: find someone or a group of people achieving the results you want to achieve. You can then discover their eating plan – once you have that you can model the plan and see if it works for you. Remember to also consider how close the "people" you are modelling are to you in body-size, shape, culture and metabolism. What's interesting is that many different cultures across the world have evolved separately to consume different diets. For instance, the Inuit in Northern Canada subsist entirely on seal meat and fat, with some additional sources of protein in the form of small birds and carbohydrates such as tubers, vegetables and leafy greens in the short summers. However, cultures in India have evolved to live long-lasting, healthy lives based entirely on diets consisting of vegetables and nuts with no dairy whatsoever.

Let's take a look at a couple of key studies in relation to diet and food consumption.

The China Study, by T. Colin Campbell Ph.D., states that (in China) "some areas have essentially no cancer or heart disease, while in other areas, they reflect up to a 100-fold increase." Coincidentally, diets in China range from entirely plant based to heavily animal-based, depending on the location. It was those areas with lower animal-based food intake that registered far lower in cancer and heart disease. In contrast, diseases of affluence such as cancer and heart disease are common throughout the United States. Most Americans eat an animal-protein based diet, with relatively few calories coming from plant foods.

The cover article of the November 2005 issue of *National Geographic* was titled "*The Secrets of LIVING LONGER*". The article opens with the sentence, "What if I said you could add up to ten years to your life?" It's basically a lifestyle survey of three populations: Sardinians, Okinawans, and Adventists. These populations generally display longevity and "suffer a fraction of the diseases that commonly kill people in other parts of the developed world, and enjoy more healthy years of life. In sum, they offer three sets of best practices to emulate. The rest is up to you."

The common tendency in all three groups is to "Eat fruits, vegetables, and whole grains." The article noted that an NIH funded study of 34,000 Seventh-Day Adventists between 1976 and 1988 "...found that the Adventists' habit of consuming beans, soy milk, tomatoes, and other fruits lowered their risk of developing certain cancers. It also suggested that eating whole wheat bread, drinking five glasses of water a day, and, most surprisingly, consuming four servings of nuts a week reduced their risk of heart disease. And it found that not eating red meat had been helpful to avoid both cancer and heart disease."

It has been discovered that people living in Southern France live longer. Even though they consume a comparable amount of saturated fats, the rate of heart disease is lower in Southern France than in North America. A number of explanations have been suggested:

- reduced consumption of processed carbohydrates and other junk foods

- regular consumption of red wine

- living in the south requires the body to produce less heat, allowing a slower, and therefore healthier, metabolic rate

- one of the other issues identified in many Mediterranean (traditional) diets and eating plans is that food tends to be acquired, prepared and eaten within a short space of time with less processed and stored foods entering the food patterns of people living within long time cultural norms

Here's one more idea to consider...

Ancient Hawaiian teachings in relation to food said that if you consume something and it makes you feel light and energetic after eating it, eat more of it. If you consume something that makes you feel enervated and lethargic afterwards – then don't eat it again. It's all about truly listening to your body.

First tip: whenever you are hungry always drink water first. Remember, hunger signals are often misinterpreted thirst signals. When you see or smell food, a hormone called ghrelin is released from your endocrine system that prepares your digestive system for the incoming meal. Drinking water instead of eating will suppress this feeling. Once you've had a good drink, waited a little while and are still hungry, then by all means eat.

Eating frequency is another very personal thing. Some people find that they are more energetic if they eat small amounts and often. Others feel completely satisfied eating one or two large meals per day, getting most of their calories at key moments. Intermittent fasting is also another aspect of diet that should be explored. If you're feeling full and satisfied and don't feel like you don't need to eat, then don't eat! Some people can go for up to 30 hours or even more without eating. A lot of athletes and those interested in working out are interested in this kind of dietary lifestyle.

Second tip: our bodies are much smarter than we are. Take note over the next week or so. How do you feel after eating what it was that you ate? Did it make you feel light and energised or did it weigh you down?

So how do we use what we know?

The process is this:

Acceptance

Once you have new information, particularly if it is different to how you have thought or operated within the past, it is critical to "accept" that there is a different way of approaching things; a potentially new and different way to do things and therefore achieve different results that could be available to you. It is also equally important to accept that you might want to change your old habits for new ones in order to reach a better result. Your diet is a personal thing and based on your culture and genetics. Explore how your ancestors ate and experiment with different types of diets and find the one that works for you. The one that is making you feel the most energetic is probably the right one. You need to accept that if something is making you feel enervated and lethargic then it might be a good idea to move on and try another type of diet until you find the right one that works for you.

Awareness

Becoming "aware" is the first (and sometimes only) thing necessary for change. It is the crucial step to changing the results. You must become aware of where your body is currently and what you need to do to change your diet to get where you want to be. Aware of the new habits to be taken in and the new possibilities that will open up to you once you begin to act in new ways.

Activation

All the "thinking" done – it's time for "*real*-ising" – that is, making it happen in the real world – and putting into action what you know you need to do. If this means giving up food sources that are bad for your health if consumed in excessive quantities, then it's a change that you will have to make in your life to achieve the results you want.

Appreciate

Finally, as in all things, it is critical to "appreciate" what you have accomplished and be grateful for having achieved it. If you're not happy with the way your body and your diet is now, then you can still appreciate that whatever you were doing was a learning experience for you. You can use your new-found knowledge to move onto a better diet and lifestyle that will bring your body back into harmony. Even if it is one step forward on a long journey you are now one step further along the path and that is infinitely better than where you were before; even accepting that there could be change. Appreciation is the step we keep with us constantly; every change, improvement and moment of growth is a moment to appreciate what you have done and what you are "doing" even now. It is important to go as far as to reward yourself for the achievements. "Celebrate All Achievements" is a mantra you can use for any aspect of your diet as well. Don't despair if you are unhealthy now, the knowledge of this fact is something you can appreciate and learn from. "Celebrate Everything", even those things that made you unhealthy at some point in the past.

Where does this leave you right now? You have read and completed the "acceptance" bit; now it's time for awareness. Think where you are currently "at" with breathing consciously and how you use this fundamental mechanism for physical success to your own advantage.

Rate yourself below on a scale of 1-10.

1: I suck at this. Through to 10: I'm incredible at this.
If you scored yourself a "4" or below, then it's time to take some massive action in this area. You need a strategy to create change here.

❶ Where are you now?

○ ○ ○ ○ ○ ○ ○ ○ ○ ○
1　2　3　4　5　6　7　8　9　10

❷ Where do you want to be in 30 days?

○ ○ ○ ○ ○ ○ ○ ○ ○ ○
1　2　3　4　5　6　7　8　9　10

❸ Where do you want to be in 3 months?

○ ○ ○ ○ ○ ○ ○ ○ ○ ○
1　2　3　4　5　6　7　8　9　10

❹ Where do you want to be in 6 months?

○ ○ ○ ○ ○ ○ ○ ○ ○ ○
1　2　3　4　5　6　7　8　9　10

❺ Where do you want to be in 12 months?

○ ○ ○ ○ ○ ○ ○ ○ ○ ○
1　2　3　4　5　6　7　8　9　10

❻ What aspects do you want to learn, change, grow, develop?

_____

_____

_____

7 How do you want to do that?

8 What impact will that have on your life and/or the lives of those you love most?

9 What is your plan? (Include names, dates, actions.)

10 The first thing I need to do to make this happen is...

11 I'm going to do this when?

12 To whom or how am I going to be held accountable...

13 Today I will...

14 **This week I will...**

_____

_____

15 **I'm ready to do this because...**

_____

_____

_____

That's it: plan set. Now it's time for you to put it in motion. If you have any work to do there, then it needs to be done and the momentum built. Do not move on to the next part until you have done something actively and positively towards shifting your personal outcome in this area. You don't have to have achieved your ultimate goal – just make sure you have a plan and that plan is already in play through your own actions.

When you are ready, let's get to the next secret. The secrets of...

5. abundance in dynamic exercise

 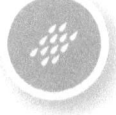     

abundance in dynamic exercise

Dynamic Exercise begins a cycle with Restful Sleep of positive dependence; one forms the foundation for the other, which in turn creates the basis for the other. It relies on physical exercise: that is the performance of some activity in order to develop or maintain physical fitness and overall health. And it is so much more than that.

It not just about honing athletic ability or skill. Frequent and regular dynamic exercise is an important component in the prevention of some of the "diseases of affluence" such as cancer, heart disease, cardiovascular disease, Type 2 diabetes and obesity.

Exercise is important for the three main areas of physical wellness: flexibility, endurance and strength. All are important.

Dynamic physical exercise is considered important for maintaining physical fitness, including healthy weight; building and maintaining healthy bones, muscles, and joints; promoting physiological well-being; reducing surgical risks; and strengthening the immune system.

The American College of Sports Medicine recommends that all people regularly do activities that address each component of overall fitness: cardiovascular endurance (achieved through aerobic activity), strength (achieved through weight-lifting) and flexibility (achieved through stretching). Each of these types of exercise can improve one's sense of psychological well-being.

Some of the physical payoffs for exercise:

- decreased resting heart rate
- improved recovery time (heart rate returns to its resting level faster)
- decreased resting blood pressure
- increased efficiency of heart (heart pumps more blood with each stroke)
- decreased muscle tension
- weight management
- increased endurance
- better quality of sleep/reduced fatigue
- better appetite regulation
- more efficient use of food energy
- increased resistance to colds & other illnesses
- decreased cholesterol and triglyceride levels
- decreased body fat/increased muscle bulk & tone
- decreased bone demineralisation
- increased tolerance to heat and cold

In the early 1980s, a neurotransmitter (a brain chemical) was discovered which showed remarkable morphine-like qualities. In very small amounts, it was found to significantly reduce sensations of pain and seemed to promote feelings of euphoria and exhilaration while reducing feelings of depression and anxiety. Because this neurotransmitter is synthesised during aerobic activity (exercise that increases your cardiovascular output – breathing and heart rate), exercise has become a major part of stress-reduction programs, pain management programs, and self-care for depression, anxiety and many other disorders.

Following are some other benefits of regular exercise, particularly aerobic activity:

- improved self-esteem
- improved sense of self-reliance, self-confidence and self-efficacy
- improved mental alertness, perception and information processing
- increased perceptions of acceptance by others
- decreased overall feelings of stress and tension
- reduced frustration with daily "hassles"
- more constructive responses to disappointments and failures

Most people readily agree that exercise is generally good for them – but how do you get started when it is not your "norm" now?

If you are currently living a more sedentary lifestyle (without much exercise, etc.), it is advisable to start slowly so that you don't get discouraged with your new exercise routine and quit before you've experienced any benefits. It is of course critical that you also seek medical advice and get checked out physically before starting any program. What you want is to improve your health and not to jump into something that will injure you and cause you to not be able to exercise due to a recovery from injury. Choose an activity that you would enjoy and stick with – walking is as good as any that requires expensive equipment.

The goal is simply to start moving more.

Start with 15 minutes every other day and gradually increase the amount of time and number of days. Thirty minutes five or six days a week is ideal, but if you are willing to do only 20 minutes four days a week, it's better than nothing at all.

The best advice anyone can get when starting to exercise is to seek professional and expert advice. First of all, your health carer – what are you currently capable of and can you do it? Secondly, from the Fitness Industry – a Personal Trainer is a major asset in achieving a level of Dynamic Physical Exercise needed to improve health and wellness. Be guided by the professionals and remember to keep your goals in mind.

So, how strenuous is enough but not too much? The best guideline is to keep your heart rate within its training zone for the entire duration of each workout. To do this, compute your maximum heart rate by subtracting your age from 220. Multiply this number first by 65% and then by 80%. This will give you a lower and upper limit for your heart rate during exercise. For people who have been sedentary for a long time or who want to maximise fat loss, keep your heart rate at the lower end of that range, around 65% to 70% of maximum.

If you don't want to mess around with heart rates, all is not lost, use your judgement. If you can't speak an intelligible sentence while exercising because you are too breathless, the activity is too strenuous. Conversely, if you are not breaking out in a light overall sweat and breathing faster than you do at rest, it's not strenuous enough. Try to find a pace that you believe you could keep up for 20-30 consecutive minutes when you are healthy. If you don't think you can keep up the pace that you've chosen, it's probably too strenuous.

What to do?

If you are searching for something to do - look for something that you can "fall in love with"; if you can do something that you LOVE — exercise and activity becomes JOYOUS.

Finally, it is said that the basis of dynamic exercise is restful sleep and the basis of a restful sleep is dynamic exercise. Exercise and Rest work hand in hand to increase your health and energy levels.

So how do we use what we know?

The process is this:

Acceptance

Once you have new information, particularly if it is different to how you have thought or operated within the past, it is critical to "accept" that there is a different way of approaching things; a potentially new and different way to do things and therefore achieve different results that could be available to you. If you've been largely sedentary for most of your life, it might be difficult to start exercising, but you need to accept that this is another important aspect of your overall well-being that you need to address. It is also equally important to accept that you might want to change your old habits for new ones in order to reach a better result.

Awareness

Becoming "aware" is the first (and sometimes only) thing necessary for change. Becoming aware of a need for abundance in exercise is a crucial step to changing the results of your health. You must become aware of where you are in your exercise levels and what you are doing to increase these. It's important to be aware of the new habits to be taken in and the new possibilities that will open up to you once you begin to act in new ways.

Activation

All the "thinking" done – it's time for "*real-*ising" – that is, making it happen in the real world – and putting into action what you know you need to do. You need to find an activity that you truly love and enjoy – whether it's taking long walks by the river, cycling, martial arts, horseback riding, calisthenics, yoga or anything else. It's not hard to do "exercise" when you're not thinking of it as exercise, but rather a hobby that's well and truly part of your lifestyle.

Appreciate

Finally, as in all things, it is critical to "appreciate" what you have accomplished and be grateful for having achieved it. It's not hard to appreciate the things you love, so pick activities that you love. What's the point in doing something you hate? You'll never appreciate it. Find a physical activity that you love and add it to your lifestyle. Even if it is one step forward on a long journey you are now one step further along the path and that is infinitely better than where you were before; even accepting that there could be change. Appreciation is the step we keep with us constantly; every change, improvement and moment of growth is a moment to appreciate what you have done and what you are "doing" even now. It is important to go as far as to reward yourself for the achievements. "Celebrate All Achievements" is not only the achievement of the goal that required reward but rather every step along the way that is begging for recognition. Abundant energy in exercise leads you inevitably to "Celebrate Everything".

Where does this leave you right now? You have read and completed the "acceptance" bit; now it's time for awareness. Think where you are currently "at" with breathing consciously and how you use this fundamental mechanism for physical success to your own advantage.

Rate yourself below on a scale of 1-10.

1: I suck at this. Through to 10: I'm incredible at this.
If you scored yourself a "4" or below, then it's time to take some massive action in this area. You need a strategy to create change here.

❶ Where are you now with regards to exercise?

○ ○ ○ ○ ○ ○ ○ ○ ○ ○
1　2　3　4　5　6　7　8　9　10

❷ Where do you want to be in 30 days? What cardio or endurance goal would you like to achieve by this time?

○ ○ ○ ○ ○ ○ ○ ○ ○ ○
1　2　3　4　5　6　7　8　9　10

❸ Where do you want to be in 3 months? What cardio or endurance goal would you like to achieve by this time?

○ ○ ○ ○ ○ ○ ○ ○ ○ ○
1　2　3　4　5　6　7　8　9　10

❹ Where do you want to be in 6 months? What cardio or endurance goal would you like to achieve by this time?

○ ○ ○ ○ ○ ○ ○ ○ ○ ○
1　2　3　4　5　6　7　8　9　10

❺ Where do you want to be in 12 months? What cardio or endurance goal would you like to achieve by this time?

○ ○ ○ ○ ○ ○ ○ ○ ○ ○
1　2　3　4　5　6　7　8　9　10

6 What aspects do you want to learn, change, grow, develop? What new sports or physical activities will you become better at?

_____
_____

7 How do you want to do that? Will you join a club? Will you spend more time with friends who are into this activity?

_____
_____

8 What impact will that have on your life and/or the lives of those you love most?

_____
_____

9 What is your plan? (Include names, dates, actions.)

_____
_____

10 The first thing I need to do to make this happen is...

_____
_____

11 I'm going to do this when?

_____
_____

12 To whom or how am I going to be held accountable...

_____
_____

13 Today I will...

_____

_____

14 This week I will...

_____

_____

15 I'm ready to do this because...

_____

_____

_____

That's it: plan set. Now it's time for you to put it in motion. If you have any work to do there, then it needs to be done and the momentum built. Do not move on to the next part until you have done something actively and positively towards shifting your personal outcome in this area. You don't have to have achieved your ultimate goal – just make sure you have a plan and that plan is already in play through your own actions.

When you are ready, let's get to the next secret. The secrets of...

6. abundance in restful sleep

abundance in restful sleep

The interplay between Dynamic Exercise and Restful Sleep is essential for Energy in Abundance. Dynamic Exercise becomes the foundation of Restful Sleep. There is not one perfect time to start; begin with either and enjoy the benefits of both. Restful Sleep helps the body restore and rejuvenate in many different ways including:

Memory, Learning and Social Processes – Sleep enables the brain to process, code and store information properly. REM sleep activates the parts of the brain that control learning. The parts of the brain that control emotions, decision-making and social interactions slow down dramatically during sleep, allowing optimal performance when awake.

Nervous System – Sleep experts now suggest the possibility that neurons used during the day repair themselves during sleep.

Immune System – Sleep also enables the immune system to function effectively. Without proper sleep, the immune system becomes weak and the body becomes more vulnerable to infection and disease.

Growth and Development – Children need much more sleep than adults. But even in adults, the growth hormone somatotropin is released during sleep, so sleep is vital to proper physical and mental development. When you do strenuous physical exercise and then spend a few days resting, your body is building stronger cells to replace the old ones that were damaged while active. It's also worth knowing that whatever you are consuming as nutrition is used by this hormone to build muscle and bone cells while you sleep. If you've ever seen or had puppies at home, you know this simply by observing their cycle and watching their bodies change. Eat, sleep, eat, sleep – and they just get bigger and bigger. It's clear to anyone that sleep and nutrition are fundamentally related, as are many of the things we should be abundant in talked about in this book.

It's also important to understand what sleep is including the stages we go through when we are sleeping. There are five stages of sleep: stages 1, 2, 3, 4 and REM (rapid eye movement).

The body cycles through the different sleep stages from stage 1 to REM and then begins again with stage 1. Each stage represents a different physical and mental state of the body during sleep.

The National Institute of Neurological Disorders and Stroke provides this description of the five sleep stages:

> Stage 1 (Drowsiness) – We drift in and out of sleep for about 5 to 10 minutes and can be awakened easily. Our eyes move very slowly and muscle activity slows.
>
> Stage 2 (Light Sleep) – Our eye movements stop and our brain waves (fluctuations of electrical activity that can be measured by electrodes) become slower, with occasional bursts of rapid waves called sleep spindles. Our heart rate slows and body temperature decreases.
>
> Stages 3 and 4 (Deep Sleep) – Slow brain waves called delta waves begin to appear, interspersed with smaller, faster waves. By Stage 4 the brain produces delta waves almost exclusively. It is very difficult to wake someone during stages 3 and 4, which together are called deep sleep. There is no eye movement or muscle activity. People awakened during deep sleep do not adjust immediately and often feel groggy and disoriented for several minutes after they wake up. Some children experience bedwetting, night terrors, or sleepwalking during these stages.

REM Sleep – During REM sleep, our breathing becomes more rapid, irregular, and shallow, our eyes jerk rapidly in various directions, and our limb muscles become temporarily paralysed. Our heart rate increases, our blood pressure rises, and males develop penile erections. People dream during this stage.

The average length of time for a complete sleep cycle is 90-110 minutes. About 50 percent of sleep time is spent in stage 2 and about 20 percent in REM sleep. The remaining 30 percent is split between the other stages. On average, a person will cycle through the stages 4 or 5 times in an eight hour period. After a person falls asleep, the first REM sleep period generally happens 70-90 minutes later.

Adequate sleep is crucial to proper brain function – no less so than air, water, and food – but stress can modify sleep-wakefulness cycles. Even a small amount of sleep deprivation will diminish mental performance, with evidence that even just one full night of sleep deprivation can be equivalent to legally intoxicated blood-alcohol levels in a controlled driving/response test.

Many people don't assess how much sleep they need for optimal functioning; they just know they don't get enough. Every person's sleep requirement is different. Some find they only need 5-6 hours of sleep, while others need 10-11 hours to be at their best. The average adult functions best with 7-8 hours of sleep a night. It's more important to consider how much sleep you need on an individual basis.

Sleep Experts have developed some guidelines to help you consider how much sleep you or your loved ones might need:

Infants and Children – Infants require about 16 hours a day. From 6 months to about 3 years, children's sleep requirement decreases to about 14 hours. Young children generally get their sleep from a combination of night-time sleep and naps.

Teenagers – Teenagers need about 9 hours of sleep a night. Sleep is crucial for teenagers because it is while they are sleeping that their bodies release the hormone somatotropin in huge amounts that is essential during their growth spurt.

Adults – For most adults, 7 to 8 hours a night appears to be the best amount of sleep, although the amount ranges from 5 hours to 10 hours of sleep each day depending on the individual. It should be noted that a recent research study conducted by Boston University School of Medicine found that study participants that reported sleeping less than 6 hours or more than 9 hours a day had an increased incidence of diabetes, compared to those who slept 7-8 hours. On the other hand, it's important to take into account the fact that some of the world's top Olympic level athletes, such as Roger Federer, Lebron James and Michelle Wie have reported that they get up to 12 hours of sleep a night. The amount of sleep you need, like diet, is highly personal and you should find out what works best for you and gives you the greatest energy levels and stick to that.

Pregnant Women – Women in the first trimester of pregnancy, and sometimes throughout pregnancy, need significantly more sleep than usual.

Some of the signs that indicate you may need more sleep include:

- difficulty waking up
- lack of concentration
- falling asleep at the wrong time, such as during class or work
- moodiness, irritability, depression or anxiety
- micro-sleeps, brief episodes of sleep during the day, are also an indication that you are sleep deprived

If you are consistently tired or drowsy during the day, you probably aren't getting enough sleep.

Getting less sleep than needed can cause a "sleep debt", meaning that your body expects to make up that missed sleep. You can make up for missed sleep during a night by sleeping more the next night, or compensate for missed sleep during the week by sleeping more on the weekend. Getting the missed sleep is important because, physically, the body needs it to recover and restore itself. Some people claim to get used to sleeping less. They may think their body adjusts to a sleep-deprived schedule, but this probably isn't the case. Generally, people who aren't getting enough sleep show mental and physical signs of sleep deprivation during their waking hours.

That's all the research and study as to why. I am sure you are at least a little convinced by how. So the question is how to improve sleep. Having coached thousands of people on improving their energy levels I have found the most common problem is lack of or poor sleep and the most wanted (and needed) assistance was with either getting more or improving the sleep they were getting. So here are my top tips for improving sleep and truly achieving the level of Restful Sleep that will impact your Energy & Abundance.

Let's start with what you are doing during the day. The foundation for your new achievement comes before you even think about getting into bed:

- **Do not nap during the day.** If you are having trouble sleeping at night, try not to nap during the day because you will throw off your body clock and make it even more difficult to sleep at night. If you are feeling especially tired, and feel as if you absolutely must get some sleep try a "Power Nap" – the ideas behind this have become more popular and accepted in recent years. Many of the greatest minds of the past and present used "Power Napping" to overcome any sleep debt incurred due to heavy work loads. Do not sleep any more than 30 minutes at a time during the day. If you are really having trouble sleeping at night – only have one "nap" during the day.

- **Limit caffeine and alcohol.** Avoid drinking caffeinated drinks or alcohol of any kind for several hours before bedtime. Although alcohol may initially act as a sedative, it can definitely interrupt normal sleep patterns.

- **Don't smoke and watch out for over the counter drugs too.** Nicotine is a stimulant and can make it difficult to fall asleep and stay asleep. Many over-the-counter and prescription drugs disrupt sleep.

- **Expose yourself to bright light/sunlight soon after awakening.** This will help to regulate your body's natural biological clock. Sunlight will dissipate the body's own "sleep chemicals" naturally (wherever possible developing energy and abundance for the long term means working with the natural processes already available to us). So, likewise, try to keep your bedroom dark while you are sleeping so that the light will not interfere with your rest.

- **Exercise early in the day.** Twenty to thirty minutes of exercise every day can help you sleep, but be sure to exercise in the morning or afternoon. Because exercise stimulates the body, activity before bedtime could make falling asleep more difficult.

- **Check your iron levels.** Iron deficient women tend to have more problems sleeping so if your blood is iron poor, a supplement might help your health and your ability to sleep.

So that's what you could do during the day. How about the bedroom (or whatever your sleeping environment is)?

- **Make sure your bed is large enough and comfortable.** If you are disturbed by a restless bed-mate, switch to a queen- or king-size bed. Test different types of mattresses. Even if you sleep by yourself more often, you need to make sure your bed is actually big enough for you to be comfortable. You can also try therapeutically-shaped foam pillows that cradle your neck (often sold by chiropractors) or extra pillows that help you sleep on your side. Also look at your bedding – you should have comfortable cotton sheets that allow your body to "breathe".

- **Make your bedroom primarily a place for sleeping.** The bedroom is a place for sleeping and "special cuddles". It is not a good idea to use your bed for paying bills, doing work, etc. Help your body recognise that this is a place for rest or intimacy. If you use your bedroom for entertainment (not in "that" way!) – meaning TV, reading etc., or bills, work and whatever else you will not develop a strong anchor to the "rest" needed in that room. TVs, etc., are best left in their rightful place in other areas of your home and not the bedroom. There are many suggestions that it is also helpful for our overall health to remove as many electrical appliances from our bedrooms.

- **Keep your bedroom peaceful and comfortable.** Make sure your room is well ventilated and the temperature consistent. And try to keep it quiet. You could use a fan or a "white noise" machine to help block outside noises. There are even apps now available on iPhones etc., that can work like "white noise" sleep machines. If using an iPhone etc., for sleep/alarm ensure its capacity for radio signals is switched off – put it on "flight mode" like on a plane.

- **Temperature in the bed is also important.** One of the primary reasons for poor sleep is the fact that once we are in bed our own body heat tends to be trapped by the bedding and even though we went to bed feeling "toasty" we soon become "roasty" and our sleep is disturbed. The best temperature level to fall asleep in is one that is comfortable but still cool – with sheets, blankets etc., your body will soon warm up the bed and you will have a much more pleasant sleep.

- **Hide your clock.** A big, illuminated digital clock may cause you to focus on the time and make you feel stressed and anxious. People who have difficulty sleeping will often wake up and look straight to the clock to count up the hours they have not been falling asleep – this only serves to enhance your anxiety for not sleeping. The body then begins to respond in any way other than becoming restful. Place your clock so you can't see the time when you are in bed. In fact, my recommendation is to get rid of the "alarm clock" all together. Whenever I get to a new hotel room the first thing I do is unplug the alarm. I prefer to use my phone (on flight mode) but keep it face down so I have to pick it up and look at the time when I need to and there is no disturbing light or blinking time announcement.

- **Make use of new technology.** This sounds a little counter to what I have said before. Let me explain – there are a number of technologies now available to help you wake at an appropriate time and also others that help you sleep more deeply. As we discussed before, sleep is actually a progression of depths of unconsciousness. The best time to wake is when the body and mind are actually closest to the conscious state. This is a "natural" waking. An application for iPhone and other "smart phones" is currently marketed that works to do just this – it is called "Sleep Cycle". I have used this for some time and find it helps me wake at the optimum time every time.

  As for getting to sleep initially – a lot of "hypnosis" style programs are also available. The best one I have used is also an application on iPhone called "Pzizz". The Pzizz device has been around for a while now – the application on iPhone is reasonably new and works very well. It is also a great aid for Power Napping due to its programmable settings.

- **Just as when we are teaching children to develop a sleep schedule through setting up "rituals", it is also important for grown ups.** Rituals prepare the unconscious mind for what is to come. In the case of improved Restful Sleep they can also create anchors to assist us in resting.

- **Keep a regular schedule.** Try to go to bed and wake up at the same time everyday, even on the weekends. Keeping a regular schedule will help your body expect sleep at the same time each day. Don't oversleep to make up for a poor night's sleep – doing that for even a couple of days can reset your body clock and make it hard for you to get to sleep at night. Paying back sleep debt is important, but do this in a day; be careful to not make a new pattern.

- **Incorporate bedtime rituals**; listening to soft music, sipping a cup of herbal tea, etc. This tells your body that it's time to slow down and begin to prepare for sleep. Hey, it worked for the kids – it will work for us too.

- **Relax for a while before going to bed.** Spending quiet time can make falling asleep easier. You can include meditation, relaxation and/or breathing exercises (all other parts of this program) or even taking a warm bath. Try listening to recorded relaxation or watch guided imagery programs; the Pzizz is also good for this.

- **Don't eat a large, heavy meal before bed.** This can cause indigestion and interfere with your normal sleep cycle. Drinking too much fluid before bed can cause you to get up to urinate. Try to eat your night meal at least two hours before you go to sleep. There are some people who even incorporate a large number of hours of fasting into their daily routine, by simply not eating for a few hours before and after they wake up. This intermittent fasting can also increase your energy levels by vast amounts, as your body quickly learns when it is time to eat and when it is time to rest and build up strength.

- **Eat more turkey.** This one has always gotten the most laughs and then when people realised I wasn't joking, the most confused stares. Well, it's not really a joke – more of an exaggeration. It doesn't have to be turkey. An amino acid called tryptophan, found in milk, turkey, and peanuts, helps the brain produce serotonin which is a natural chemical that helps you relax. Try drinking warm milk or eat a slice of toast with peanut butter or a bowl of cereal before bedtime. Plus, the warmth may temporarily increase your body temperature and the subsequent drop may hasten sleep. There was some wisdom in those old tales about milk and cookies after all...

It's important to understand that these types of measures work for many, but not all people. Just as we've discovered and discussed for diet, all people are different and work incredibly differently. What would work to send one person to sleepy-land may not work for another. For some, food keeps them awake; particularly anything containing sugars (such as milk, breads or other cereals). Someone in this category could try using the intermittent fasting techniques spoken about earlier. The answer is – if what you are doing isn't working for YOU, then try something else.

- **Keep a journal or notepad beside your bed.** Jot down all of your concerns and worries. Anxiety excites and disturbs the nervous system, so your brain sends messages to the adrenal glands, making you more alert. When you write down your worries and possible solutions before you go to bed, you don't need to ruminate in the middle of the night. A journal or "to-do" list may be very helpful in letting you put away these concerns until the next day when you are fresh. Many people will wake from sleep to worry about things for the next day as well – having the book or pad right there lets you get the ideas "out of your head and onto paper" so you can get to worry about them tomorrow without forgetting. This means you can get back to sleep now.

- **Go to sleep when you are sleepy.** When you feel tired, go to bed. Many people just "do one more thing" or "read one more page" or "watch till the next ad break". Don't. The best time for you to sleep is when you are tired. Take your body's word for it and get to bed while you can. If you miss this window you might have to wait 45–90 minutes for the next cycle of alertness to tiredness to come around.

- **Avoid "over-the-counter" sleep aids**, and make sure that your prescribed medications do not cause insomnia. There is little evidence that many supplements and other over-the-counter "sleep aids" are effective. In some cases, there are safety concerns. Antihistamine sleep aids, in particular, have a long duration of action and can cause daytime drowsiness. Always talk to your doctor or healthcare practitioner about your concerns.

So you've done good during the day, got the sleep area sorted and gone through your rituals – what if you wake up during the night – what then?

- **Do visualisation.** Focus all your attention on your toes or visualise walking down an endless stairwell. Thinking about repetitive or mindless things will help your brain to shut down and adjust to sleep. You can also use what hypnotists call "deepening techniques". Visualise and imagine being on a calm beach and letting the waves wash over your feet with each successive wave washing in relaxation and away your "alertness" or try walking down stairs etc., with each step bringing you more relaxation till you find a bed at the bottom and curl up in it to sleep.

- **Get out of bed if unable to sleep.** Don't lie in bed awake; so many people toss and turn in their beds awake and totally unable to go back to sleep. This is because restfulness and readiness to sleep are cyclical. Instead of lying there and proving to yourself you cannot go back to sleep simply get up and do something else till you get tired again. Go into another room and do something relaxing until you feel sleepy. Worrying about falling asleep actually keeps many people awake. When Milton Erickson (called the "Father of Modern Hypnosis") worked with people having difficulty getting back to sleep he could get them to wake up, get up and do the most unpleasant chores they could think of. Then when tired enough they'd simply go back to bed and sleep.

- **Don't do anything stimulating.** Don't read anything job-related or watch a stimulating TV program (commercials and news shows tend to be alerting). Don't expose yourself to bright light. The light gives cues to your brain that it is time to wake up. Of course you don't have your TV in your bedroom anymore anyway... right? There are also a number of great applications available for your computer which will dim the monitor based on the time of day and change its base colour slightly as well so if you are working late at a computer, your eyes will not suffer from glare too much when it's dark outside. These programs have been shown to improve sleep patterns as well.

- **Consider changing your bedtime.** If you are experiencing sleeplessness or insomnia consistently, think about going to bed later so that the time you spend in bed is spent sleeping. If you are only getting five hours of sleep at night, figure out what time you need to get up and subtract five hours (for example, if you want to get up at 6:00 am, go to bed at 1:00 am). This may seem counterproductive and, at first, you may be depriving yourself of some sleep, but it can help train your body to sleep consistently while in bed. When you are spending all of your time in bed sleeping, you can gradually sleep more, by adding 15 minutes at a time.

And when all else fails...

- **Get up and eat some turkey... no joke!** Remember, turkey contains tryptophan, a major building block for making serotonin, a neurotransmitter, which sends messages between nerve cells and causes feelings of sleepiness. Eating foods containing tryptophan raise the levels of serotonin produced in the body, which in turn increases a person's feeling of sleepiness. It is best to eat tryptophan on an empty stomach. You can also find a good amount of tryptophan in milk, cottage cheese, yoghurt, ice cream, chicken, cashews, soy beans, tuna and of course... turkey.

So how do we use what we know?

The process is this:

Acceptance

Once you have new information about sleep and sleep patterns, particularly if it is different to how you have thought about sleep in the past, it is critical to "accept" that there is a different way of approaching things; you may need to accept that you are not getting enough sleep every night or that you may even be sleeping too much. It is also equally important to accept that you might want to change your old habits for new ones in order to reach a better result.

Awareness

Becoming "aware" is the first (and sometimes only) thing necessary for change. Become aware that you either need more or less sleep and you will take that first crucial step to changing the results. You must become aware of where you are at and what you are doing with your sleep patterns. Also be aware of the new habits to be taken in and the new possibilities that will open up to you once you begin to act in new ways.

Activation

All the "thinking" done – it's time for "*real-*ising" – that is, making it happen in the real world – and putting into action what you know you need to do. Use blinds to make your bedroom dark, remove electrical appliances, increase or decrease the amount of hours you sleep, get plenty of water and sunlight when you wake up, and so on.

Appreciate

Finally, as in all things, it is critical to "appreciate" what you have accomplished and be grateful for having achieved it. It's not hard to appreciate your new sleep patterns once you realise that you are full of energy and never tired again! Even if it is one step forward on a long journey, because you added 15 minutes to your deficient sleep time, you are still now one step further along the path and that is infinitely better than where you were before; even accepting that there could be change. Appreciation is the step we keep with us constantly; every change, improvement and moment of growth is a moment to appreciate what you have done and what you are "doing" even now. It is important to go as far as to reward yourself for the achievements. "Celebrate All Achievements" is a motto that can easily change into "Celebrate Everything", when you realise that every step of your journey begs for recognition and reward.

Where does this leave you right now? You have read and completed the "acceptance" bit; now it's time for awareness. Think where you are currently "at" with breathing consciously and how you use this fundamental mechanism for physical success to your own advantage.

Rate yourself below on a scale of 1-10.

1: I suck at this. Through to 10: I'm incredible at this.
If you scored yourself a "4" or below, then it's time to take some massive action in this area. You need a strategy to create change here.

❶ Where are you now? How much are you sleeping every night?
○ ○ ○ ○ ○ ○ ○ ○ ○ ○
1   2   3   4   5   6   7   8   9   10

❷ Where do you want to be in 30 days? How much sleep would you like to be getting?
○ ○ ○ ○ ○ ○ ○ ○ ○ ○
1   2   3   4   5   6   7   8   9   10

❸ Where do you want to be in 3 months? How much sleep would you like to be getting?
○ ○ ○ ○ ○ ○ ○ ○ ○ ○
1   2   3   4   5   6   7   8   9   10

❹ Where do you want to be in 6 months? How much sleep would you like to be getting?
○ ○ ○ ○ ○ ○ ○ ○ ○ ○
1   2   3   4   5   6   7   8   9   10

❺ Where do you want to be in 12 months? How much sleep would you like to be getting?

○ ○ ○ ○ ○ ○ ○ ○ ○ ○
1   2   3   4   5   6   7   8   9   10

❻ What aspects do you want to learn, change, grow, develop?

_____

_____

❼ How do you want to do that?

_____

_____

❽ What impact will that have on your life and/or the lives of those you love most?

_____

_____

❾ What is your plan? (Include names, dates, actions.)

_____

_____

❿ The first thing I need to do to make this happen is...

_____

_____

⓫ I'm going to do this when?

_____

_____

⑫ To whom or how am I going to be held accountable...

_____

_____

⑬ Today I will...

_____

_____

⑭ This week I will...

_____

_____

⑮ I'm ready to do this because...

_____

_____

That's it: plan set. Now it's time for you to put it in motion. If you have any work to do there, then it needs to be done and the momentum built. Do not move on to the next part until you have done something actively and positively towards shifting your personal outcome in this area. You don't have to have achieved your ultimate goal – just make sure you have a plan and that plan is already in play through your own actions.

When you are ready, let's get to the next secret. The secrets of...

7. abundance in clear and centred mind

abundance in clear and centred mind

With the major physical conditions enabling energy and abundance handled (or well on their way) it's time to turn inward – to clearing and centring the mind. Anxiety and stress eat away at our levels of energy and abundance more so than most other things in our life. They not only contribute to many peoples' deficiencies in these areas, but they are also responsible for disabling the important physical conditions we've been working on. Meditation was for a long time (in the western world) something of a "woo woo" experimental pseudo cult-religion thing... Of course in the Eastern World and in many traditional cultures (who each have their own styles of meditation practice or behaviours) it has been a standard part of life for millennia.

In recent years there has been a growing interest within the western medical community to study the physiological effects of Meditation. It has now (for the most part) entered the mainstream of health care as a method of anxiety, stress and pain reduction. For example, in an early study reported in Scientific American in 1972, transcendental meditation was shown to affect the human metabolism by lowering the biochemical by-products of stress, such as lactate, decreasing heart rate and blood pressure, as well as inducing favourable brain waves.

As a method of stress reduction, meditation is used now in many hospitals for cases of chronic or terminal illness to reduce complications associated with increased stress including a depressed immune system. Dr. James Austin, a neurophysiologist at the University of Colorado, reported that Zen meditation rewires the circuitry of the brain in his landmark book *Zen and the Brain* (Austin, 1999). This has been confirmed using functional MRI imaging which examine the electrical activity of the brain.

The host of biochemical and physical changes in the body that have been studied during mediation are sometimes now collectively referred to as the "relaxation response" (Lazar *et. al.*, 2003). This includes changes in metabolism, heart rate, respiration, blood pressure and brain chemistry. Clinical studies have also been carried out at Buddhist monasteries in the Himalayan Mountains and on the effects of "Mindfulness Meditation" on stress levels.

But as with all health-related issues, prevention is often the best cure in the first place. Reducing stress is certainly not the only reason to meditate. Meditation is also possible as part of a lifestyle and this is how it is used in eastern practices. Actually, the reasons for which people meditate vary almost as much as practices. Meditation can be simply a means of relaxation from a busy daily routine; or a technique for cultivating mental discipline; or a way of gaining insight into the nature of reality, or even communing with one's God. Prayer can also be interpreted as a form of meditation; ask any rabbi, priest, imam, monk or minister. Regardless of the reason, many practitioners report improved concentration, awareness, self-discipline and improved life through meditation.

Many religious or spiritual based meditation practices re-enforce the need for structure and the "spiritual-centric" orientation of the "meditation sessions". I prefer a more balanced approach and what I think is potentially a more accessible one to many. When the mind is clear from chatter (that internal voice constantly talking to you – and if you just asked "which voice?" it was that one!)... a "meditative state" has been achieved. There may be times when new understandings or even moments or revelation are apparent during these periods or perhaps it is just a time for quiet and peace. Either way this is of great benefit.

The one thing I know for certain about meditation is that it cannot be experienced by proxy. What is important is to do it – be in the moment and experience then make judgement as to have to use it for yourself.

Some very accessible reading on meditation and perhaps some further exploration for you can be found here: *The Miracle of Mindfulness : A Manual on Meditation*, by Thich Nhat Hanh, et al.

Whatever it is you choose, if you find yourself in need of some more clarity of mind, more peace or reduction in stress and anxiety, it is time to begin some intentional meditation.

So how do we use what we know?

The process is this:

Acceptance

Particularly if this information about mediation and a clear and centred mind is different to how you have thought or operated within the past, it is critical to "accept" that this is a new and different way of approaching things and therefore a new way to achieve different results that could be available to you. It is also equally important to accept that you might want to change your old habits for new ones in order to reach a better result.

Awareness

Becoming "aware" is the first (and sometimes only) thing necessary for change. It is the crucial step to changing the results. You must become aware of where you are and whether or not you have a clear and centred mind. Aware of the new habits to be taken in and the new possibilities that will open up to you once you begin to act in new ways.

Activation

All the "thinking" done – it's time for "*real*-ising" – that is, making it happen in the real world – and putting into action what you know you need to do. Consider adding a small meditation, prayer or other "quiet time" to your life every day. This can be 15 minutes before you go to sleep, or directly after you wake up. Be thankful and accepting of all you have and grateful for the new day. As with my book "The 7 Minute Secrets", you can also smile as soon as you wake up and clear your mind.

Appreciate

Finally, as in all things, it is critical to "appreciate" what you have accomplished and be grateful for having achieved it. Even if it is one step forward on a long journey you are now one step further along the path and that is infinitely better than where you were before; even accepting that there could be change. Appreciation for everything you have and clearing and centring your mind every day when you wake up is the crucial step to keep with us constantly; every change, improvement and moment of growth is a moment to appreciate what you have done and what you are "doing" even now. It is important to go as far as to reward yourself for the achievements. Clinton Swaine, used to teach his classes to "Celebrate All Achievements", but now he teaches his students, "Celebrate Everything", because every step of the road is worth celebrating and rewarding.

Where does this leave you right now? You have read and completed the "acceptance" bit; now it's time for awareness. Think where you are currently "at" with breathing consciously and how you use this fundamental mechanism for physical success to your own advantage.

Rate yourself below on a scale of 1-10.

1: I suck at this. Through to 10: I'm incredible at this.
If you scored yourself a "4" or below, then it's time to take some massive action in this area. You need a strategy to create change here.

❶ Where are you now? Are you meditating at all? Is your mind clear and centred?

○ ○ ○ ○ ○ ○ ○ ○ ○ ○
1 2 3 4 5 6 7 8 9 10

❷ Where do you want to be in 30 days?

○ ○ ○ ○ ○ ○ ○ ○ ○ ○
1 2 3 4 5 6 7 8 9 10

❸ Where do you want to be in 3 months?

○ ○ ○ ○ ○ ○ ○ ○ ○ ○
1 2 3 4 5 6 7 8 9 10

❹ Where do you want to be in 6 months?

○ ○ ○ ○ ○ ○ ○ ○ ○ ○
1 2 3 4 5 6 7 8 9 10

❺ Where do you want to be in 12 months?

○ ○ ○ ○ ○ ○ ○ ○ ○ ○
1 2 3 4 5 6 7 8 9 10

❻ What aspects do you want to learn, change, grow, develop?

_____

_____

7 How do you want to do that? Will you read about mediation practices? Will you start attending a religious institution or consulting with a spiritualist you trust more?

8 What impact will that have on your life and/or the lives of those you love most?

9 What is your plan? (Include names, dates, actions.)

10 The first thing I need to do to make this happen is...

11 I'm going to do this when?

12 To whom or how am I going to be held accountable.

13 Today I will...

14 This week I will...

_____

_____

15 I'm ready to do this because...

_____

_____

_____

That's it: plan set. Now it's time for you to put it in motion. If you have any work to do there, then it needs to be done and the momentum built. Do not move on to the next part until you have done something actively and positively towards shifting your personal outcome in this area. You don't have to have achieved your ultimate goal – just make sure you have a plan and that plan is already in play through your own actions.

When you are ready, let's get to the next secret. The secrets of...

8. abundance in supportive environment

 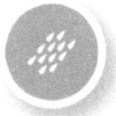     

abundance in supportive environment

I heard an analogy once about a sick fish... no matter what you do to the fish inside or out; if the water and tank are dirty and polluted you will never get it well – you have to change the water and scrub the tank. Get the environment clean. And it is the same for us. All the physical and mental (and spiritual work) we do is important and just as critical is to get our environment ready to help us maintain and even enhance the changes we've made in and out.

There are many practices that are used to create and enhance a supportive environment made up of vibrant energy and abundance. We are going to look at three major aspects:

- *Feng shui* – for your physical environment
- Time Management
- Personal Organisation & Organisers

Feng shui (pronounced "fung shway") is the ancient Chinese practice of placement and arrangement of space to achieve harmony with the environment. The literal translation is "wind and water". *Feng shui* is not just a new age decorating style.

Feng shui developed as a Chinese belief system involving a mix of many learning disciplines including geography, religion, philosophy, mathematics, aesthetics, and astrology.

According to practitioners, for a place to have "good *feng shui*" is for it to be in harmony with nature and to have "bad *feng shui*" is to be incongruous with nature. People are not classed this way but the effects of *Feng shui* are felt by all who are in the differing environments.

It was only late in the last century that information about *feng shui* began to become more widely available in the west. Before then even very little written, authoritative Chinese texts existed describing *feng shui*. Knowledge was traditionally passed down orally, but it was also believed practitioners and practice was to be intuitive and derivable from common sense and our feeling of what is natural.

In the 19th century, the Chinese government regularly published almanacs containing all the charts, diagrams, and numerical data used in *feng shui* practice.

The goal of *feng shui* guidelines is to orient dwellings, possessions, land and landscaping, etc., so as to be attuned with the flow of Qi (Life Force energy).

Very generally, some common rules are:

- When sitting at a desk or lying in bed, the entrance door should be in a clear line of sight, and you should have a view of as much of the room as possible.
- Straight lines and sharp corners are to be avoided, and especially should not point where people tend to sit, stand, or sleep.
- Avoid clutter.
- Some objects are believed to have the power of redirecting, reflecting, or shifting energy in a space. These include mirrors, crystals, wind chimes, and flowing water.

There are many wonderful books, programs and practitioners readily available all over the world now and the effects of *feng shui* again (like meditation) must be experienced first hand.

At the heart of time management is an important shift in focus: Concentrate on results, not on being busy.

Many people spend their days in a frenzy of activity, but achieve very little because they are not concentrating on the right things. When we shift focus from "doing tasks" to achieving results the actual results are almost miraculous.

One of the biggest mistakes often made by the super-busy is that they do not as Stephen Covey says, "put first things, first". His books are inspirational and paradigm shifting for many people who read them. I recommend the following to start:

- *First Things First*
- *The 7 Habits of Highly Effective People*

They are also available in audio versions and in various live trainings given by the Franklin Covey organisation or by its licensed facilitators.

Some guidelines for improving Time Management:

- Concentrate on your goals rather than the steps to get there initially; keep the goal or objective as the North Star to guide you in the right direction.
- Be flexible with what needs to be done in order to achieve the goal – not rigid in that it has to be done "your way" – this limits your responsiveness and locks you in rather than allowing you to perhaps find a more effective way (that could also be more efficient.
- Choose each month the values focus for the month. Values are like the "performance indicators for your life". Achieving them allows you to feel as though "life is good" and the opposite is true if you do not achieve

them. Decide how you will know how this month will be great for you and plan your results to help you achieve this.

- Much of what we fill our lives with is responding to urgency and unimportant items (interruptions). It is critical to determine what is truly important and to concentrate on these areas – this is the basis for Covey's work – I really encourage you to get his books (above) and work through them.

- *The 80:20 Rule* – this is neatly summed up in the Pareto Principle, or the '80:20 Rule'. This argues that typically 80% of unfocussed effort generates only 20% of results. The remaining 80% of results are achieved with only 20% of the effort. Now, the ratio is not always 80:20, but this broad pattern of a small proportion of activity generating a disproportionate result recurs so frequently as to be the norm in many areas. Are you working on the 80% or the 20%?

- In a world where it is becoming increasingly easier to delegate tasks to others and utilise currency-conversion efficiencies to do it more effectively than ever before it is important that we also realise we simply don't have to do it all ourselves. A simple rule of thumb for internal or outsourced delegation – if someone can do something 80% as well as you – delegate. You can always train the additional 20% improvement if necessary and remembering the Pareto Principle it might not even come to that.

- Personal Organisers – we all lead busy lives juggling work, family, home, and our personal interests. By organising your work and home environment, you will restore order and peace of mind into your life. You have more time to do the things you enjoy.

What does a Personal or Professional Organiser do? The National Association of Professional Organisers (NAPO) defines a Professional Organiser, as follows:

"A professional organizer employs the principles of organizing to enhance the lives of clients through the design of systems and processes. A professional organizer also educates the public on organizing solutions and the resulting benefits. A Professional Organizer takes an objective look at your organizing challenge and can provide ideas, information, systems and solutions to increase your productivity, relieve your stress and frustrations, and restore order and peace of mind into your life."

Personal Organisers have the perspective of seeing your situation with new eyes and not being bound to your previous beliefs or structures. They are also trained in leveraging the best results for you by identifying the inefficiencies in your systems (or lack of systems) and processes that you might never have imagined there.

Local business directories or professional organizer organisations in your area are the best way to get in touch with someone to help you.

- Environment, a supportive one, serves to do just that – support the changes you have made through this program. It is a critical element in cementing the transformation and not just creating transitory change.

So how do we use what we know?

The process is this:

Acceptance

Once you have new information, particularly if it is different to how you have thought or operated within the past, it is critical to "accept" that there is a different way of approaching things. In this day and age, by using the Internet and outsourcing, you can often do tasks much more efficiently by hiring virtual assistants and other professionals to do things for you more expeditiously. For many people, this is a potentially new and different way to do things and could therefore achieve different results than you experienced before. It is also equally important to accept that you might want to change your old habits for new ones in order to reach a better result; you don't have to do everything by yourself!

Awareness

Becoming "aware" is the first (and sometimes only) thing necessary for change. It is the crucial step to changing the results. You must become aware of what you can realistically do by yourself and whether or not you need to get others to help you. Become aware of the environment you are in and make changes where necessary. Become aware of the new habits to be taken in and the new possibilities that will open up to you once you begin to act in new ways.

Activation

All the "thinking" done – it's time for "*real*-ising" – that is, making it happen in the real world – and putting into action what you know you need to do. Hire an interior decorator, do it yourself, organise your time or have someone organise it for you by hiring a virtual assistant. Keep the Pareto Principle in mind and make time for all the things you love to do by hiring others to help you in your endeavours.

Appreciate

Finally, as in all things, it is critical to "appreciate" what you have accomplished and be grateful for having achieved it. Always appreciate the people you work with and give thanks for them every day. Appreciate that your environment is important and should be beautiful and relaxing for you to do the things you want to do. Even if this appreciation is only one step forward on a long journey, you are now one step further along the path and that is infinitely better than where you were before; even accepting that there could be change. Appreciation is the step we keep with us constantly; every change, improvement and moment of growth is a moment to appreciate what you have done and what you are "doing" even now. And don't forget to reward yourself for the achievements. Don't just "Celebrate All Achievements", "Celebrate Everything".

Where does this leave you right now? You have read and completed the "acceptance" bit; now it's time for awareness. Think where you are currently "at" with breathing consciously and how you use this fundamental mechanism for physical success to your own advantage.

Rate yourself below on a scale of 1-10.

1: I suck at this. Through to 10: I'm incredible at this.
If you scored yourself a "4" or below, then it's time to take some massive action in this area. You need a strategy to create change here. Where are you now? Is your space relaxing? Is your environment suitable for what you want to do?

❶ Where do you want to be in 30 days?

○ ○ ○ ○ ○ ○ ○ ○ ○ ○
1 2 3 4 5 6 7 8 9 10

❷ Where do you want to be in 3 months?

○ ○ ○ ○ ○ ○ ○ ○ ○ ○
1 2 3 4 5 6 7 8 9 10

❸ Where do you want to be in 6 months?

○ ○ ○ ○ ○ ○ ○ ○ ○ ○
1 2 3 4 5 6 7 8 9 10

❹ Where do you want to be in 12 months?

○ ○ ○ ○ ○ ○ ○ ○ ○ ○
1 2 3 4 5 6 7 8 9 10

❺ What aspects do you want to learn, change, grow, develop?

_____
_____

❻ How do you want to do that?

_____
_____

❼ What impact will that have on your life and/or the lives of those you love most?

_____
_____

❽ What is your plan? (Include names, dates, actions.)

_____
_____

❾ The first thing I need to do to make this happen is...

_____
_____

⑩ I'm going to do this when?

_____

_____

⑪ To whom or how am I going to be held accountable...

_____

_____

⑫ Today I will...

_____

_____

⑬ This week I will...

_____

_____

⑭ I'm ready to do this because...

_____

_____

That's it: plan set. Now it's time for you to put it in motion. If you have any work to do there, then it needs to be done and the momentum built. Do not move on to the next part until you have done something actively and positively towards shifting your personal outcome in this area. You don't have to have achieved your ultimate goal – just make sure you have a plan and that plan is already in play through your own actions.

When you are ready, let's get to the next secret. The secrets of...

9. conclusion

 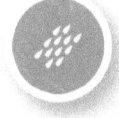     

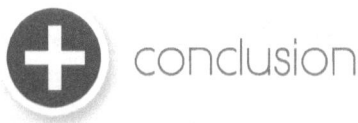

conclusion

That's it – program done! Well at least the book is.

If you have just read this straight through without taking time to do the exercises then you've been reading a lot. It really is time to DO something about it. Power is your ability to create the result you want and power will not come from knowledge alone. You must do something.

By learning, exploring or realising you have improved your mindset for change. Mindset without action is useless – nothing happens other than you will get frustrated as you know more and are not achieving more. Action is necessary to get results. Here lies a trap as well though – Action without Strategy (a plan) is wasted. If you don't know where you are heading that's exactly where you'll end up is a well known sentiment in many books and classes. To achieve a results requires 5 things:

Know what you want.

Know you can have it.

Know a plan to get it.

NOW take action.

And of course – celebrate not only your results but every step along the way.

If you have done the work along the way – BRILLIANT – please make sure you continue your changes and achievements. Keep growing and exploring and listening to your own guidance and internal wisdom as to what brings you more energy and abundance.

If you did not do the exercises and you are about to (or were thinking about it) – get on it and get on it now – it is the only way you will achieve the results.

Either way – I would love to hear about your successes and celebrations – please feel free to always send through your own stories to success@duanealley.com. If you would prefer these stories kept private, let me know. Otherwise, I would love to share them with the world so that they can celebrate you and your results as well and possibly you can help inspire others to achieve the same.

Whatever you want is out there and waiting for you.

On your way to achieving it if you are on the path anyway you might as well make it Green Lights at every turn.

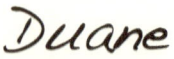

Duane Alley
Creator/Author, The 7 Secrets Series
The 7 Minute Secrets
The 7 Secrets of Energy & Abundance
7 Secret Habits of Success

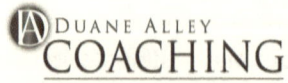

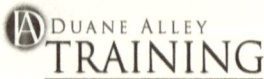

notes

notes

notes

notes

notes

notes

www.ingramcontent.com/pod-product-compliance
Lightning Source LLC
Chambersburg PA
CBHW022019290426
44109CB00015B/1231